Diabetic symptoms

General informative guide on diabetic types and how to get rid of the disease

Dr walt wade

Contents

Chapter1

introduction to diabetic mellitus

Diabetes mellitus, commonly known as diabetes, is a chronic metabolic condition that affects millions of people worldwide. According to the World Health Organization (WHO), there are currently over 422 million people living with diabetes, making it one of the most prevalent health conditions globally. This number is expected to rise to 642 million by 2040 if current trends continue. Diabetes is a leading cause of death and disability, with an estimated 1.6 million deaths directly attributed to diabetes each year. Diabetes mellitus is a condition characterized by high levels of glucose (sugar) in the blood. This is caused by the body's inability to produce enough insulin or to use it effectively. Insulin is a hormone produced by the pancreas that regulates the amount of glucose in the blood. When the body does not produce enough insulin or is resistant to its effects, excess glucose builds up in the blood, leading to high blood sugar levels. There are two main types of diabetes mellitus – type 1 and type 2. Type 1 diabetes, formerly known as juvenile diabetes, is an autoimmune condition in which the body's immune system attacks and destroys the insulin-producing cells in the pancreas. This results in little to no insulin production, requiring individuals with type 1 diabetes to take insulin for the rest of their lives. Type 1 diabetes is usually diagnosed in childhood or adolescence and accounts for about 5-10% of all diabetes cases. Type 2 diabetes, on the other hand, is a result of a combination of genetic, lifestyle, and environmental factors. In type 2 diabetes, the body is unable to use insulin effectively, a condition known as insulin resistance. This leads to high blood sugar levels, which, over time, can cause damage to various organs and tissues in the body. Type 2 diabetes is the most common form of diabetes, accounting for about 90-95% of all diabetes cases. It is more prevalent in adults, but the number of children and adolescents diagnosed with type 2 diabetes is also increasing due to rising rates of childhood obesity. One of the key risk factors for developing type 2 diabetes is being overweight or obese. A sedentary lifestyle and unhealthy eating habits can lead to weight gain, which can increase the body's resistance to insulin. Other risk factors include a family history of diabetes, ethnicity (African Americans, Hispanic/Latino Americans, Native Americans, and Asian Americans are at higher risk), and age (being over 45 years old). However, it is essential to note that not everyone with these risk factors will develop diabetes, and there may be other contributing factors as well. One of the concerning aspects of diabetes is that it often goes undiagnosed. Many people may have elevated blood sugar levels for years before they are diagnosed with diabetes, as the symptoms may be vague or absent. The most common symptoms of diabetes include frequent urination, excessive thirst, hunger, unexplained weight loss, fatigue, blurred vision, slow-healing wounds, and recurrent infections. However, these symptoms may not be noticeable in the early stages of the disease, and they may be attributed to other causes, making diabetes difficult to diagnose. If left untreated, diabetes can lead to serious health complications, including heart disease, stroke, blindness, kidney disease, nerve damage, and amputations. Therefore, early diagnosis and proper management of diabetes are crucial in preventing or delaying these complications and improving the quality of life for individuals with diabetes. The diagnosis of diabetes is made through blood tests that measure the levels of glucose in the blood. A fasting plasma glucose test measures blood glucose levels after fasting for at least 8 hours. An oral glucose tolerance test is also used, where blood glucose levels are measured before and 2 hours after consuming a glucose-rich drink. Another test used to diagnose diabetes is the glycated hemoglobin (HbA1c) test, which measures the average blood glucose levels over the past 2-3 months. Managing diabetes involves a combination of lifestyle modifications, medication, and regular monitoring of blood sugar levels. The primary goal of diabetes management is to keep blood sugar levels within a target range to prevent short-term and long-term complications. Healthy eating habits, regular physical activity, and maintaining a healthy weight are key components of managing diabetes. For individuals with type 1 diabetes, frequent blood sugar monitoring and insulin injections are necessary. In type 2 diabetes, oral medications or insulin injections may be prescribed, depending on the individual's needs. Diabetes is a significant burden not only on individuals but also on healthcare systems and economies. Its prevalence is increasing, and the impact of diabetes on individuals and society is significant. Therefore, there is a growing need for effective prevention and management strategies to control the diabetes epidemic. In conclusion, diabetes mellitus is a chronic condition characterized by high blood sugar levels caused by the body's inability to produce enough insulin or use it effectively. It has become a global health concern, with millions of people living with the disease and many more at risk of developing it. Early diagnosis, proper management, and lifestyle modifications are vital in preventing or delaying the complications associated with diabetes. It is crucial to raise awareness about diabetes and promote healthy lifestyles to reduce the burden of this disease on individuals, families, and society as a whole.

chapter2

diabetic mellitus symptoms

There are two main types of diabetes – type 1 and type 2. Type 1 diabetes is an autoimmune disorder where the body's immune system attacks and destroys the cells in the pancreas responsible for producing insulin. Type 2 diabetes, on the other hand, is a progressive condition where the body becomes resistant to the effects of insulin. The prevalence of diabetes mellitus has been increasing globally over the past few decades, with the World Health Organization (WHO) estimating that around 422 million adults were living with diabetes in 2014. The most commonly reported symptoms of diabetes mellitus include excessive thirst, frequent urination, and increased hunger. However, there are several other symptoms that are associated with this condition, and it is essential to be aware of them in order to detect and manage diabetes early on. One of the first signs of diabetes mellitus is excessive thirst or polydipsia. This is caused by the body's attempt to flush out excess glucose from the blood by increased urination. As a result, the person feels dehydrated, and the body's natural response is to crave more fluids. This excessive thirst can be persistent and difficult to quench, no matter how much water or other liquids the person drinks. Another common symptom of diabetes is frequent urination or polyuria. This is closely associated with excessive thirst, as the body tries to get rid of excess glucose by producing larger amounts of urine. People with diabetes may find themselves waking up multiple times during the night to use the bathroom. This can lead to disrupted sleep patterns and fatigue during the day. One of the classic symptoms of diabetes is increased hunger or polyphagia. In this condition, the body's cells are unable to receive glucose efficiently due to a lack of insulin or insulin resistance. This leads to a constant feeling of hunger, even after eating a sufficient amount of food. The body's cells are not getting the necessary energy from glucose, so the brain signals the body to eat more in order to meet its energy needs. Unintentional weight loss is another potential symptom of diabetes mellitus, especially in type 1 diabetes. As the body is unable to use glucose for energy, it turns to other sources such as muscle and fat. This leads to unexplained weight loss despite a proper diet and eating larger amounts of food. However, in type 2 diabetes, weight gain may occur due to insulin resistance and metabolic changes in the body. Fatigue and weakness are common symptoms of diabetes, especially in people with uncontrolled blood sugar levels. As the cells are not receiving enough glucose for energy, the body may feel fatigued and weak. This can also be caused by the body's inability to process and transport glucose to the cells, leading to a lack of energy for basic bodily functions. People with diabetes may also experience blurred vision as a symptom. High blood sugar levels can cause changes in the shape of the lens in the eye, affecting vision. If left untreated, this can lead to long-term complications such as diabetic retinopathy, which can cause permanent vision loss. Another symptom of diabetes is slow healing of wounds. High blood sugar levels can damage the blood vessels, reducing blood flow to certain areas of the body and impairing the body's natural healing process. This can lead to slow healing of cuts and bruises, as well as increased risk of infections. Some other symptoms of diabetes mellitus include dry, itchy skin, recurring infections, and tingling or numbness in the hands and feet. This can be due to damage to the nerves and blood vessels caused by high blood sugar levels. Numbness or tingling in the extremities can also be a sign of undiagnosed diabetes and should be brought to the attention of a healthcare professional. In some cases, diabetes can also lead to mood swings and irritability. Fluctuations in blood sugar levels can affect the brain's function and lead to changes in mood and behavior. It is important to monitor blood sugar levels and seek medical attention if these symptoms persist.

diabitic mellitus causes

There are several factors that can contribute to the development of diabetes, including lifestyle choices, genetics, and certain medical conditions. In this essay, we will explore the various causes of diabetes mellitus and how they contribute to the development of this chronic disease. One of the main causes of diabetes mellitus is a sedentary lifestyle. In today's modern society, people are becoming increasingly inactive due to sedentary jobs, lack of physical activity, and an abundance of processed and high-calorie foods. This sedentary lifestyle leads to obesity, which is a significant risk factor for developing Type 2 diabetes. Excess body fat, especially around the waist, can cause the body to become resistant to insulin. This means that the body's cells are unable to respond to insulin effectively, leading to high levels of glucose in the blood. Genetics also play a crucial role in the development of diabetes mellitus. Studies have shown that if one or both parents have diabetes, their offspring has a higher risk of developing the disease. However, it is not just one specific gene that causes diabetes, but a combination of genetic variations that can increase the risk. Additionally, ethnicity can also be a contributing factor. People of South Asian, African, and Hispanic descent are more likely to develop diabetes than

Caucasians. Another significant cause of diabetes mellitus is poor diet and nutrition. Consuming a diet high in processed and sugary foods can increase the risk of developing Type 2 diabetes. These foods cause a rapid rise in blood sugar levels, which puts a strain on the body's insulin production. Over time, this can lead to insulin resistance and, eventually, Type 2 diabetes. Similarly, a diet lacking in essential nutrients, such as fruits and vegetables, can also contribute to diabetes. These nutrients are essential for maintaining a healthy weight, balancing blood sugar levels, and supporting the body's use of insulin. In addition to lifestyle choices and genetics, certain medical conditions can also increase the risk of developing diabetes mellitus. One such condition is polycystic ovary syndrome (PCOS), a hormonal disorder that affects approximately one in ten women of childbearing age. Women with PCOS have higher levels of insulin in their blood, which can lead to insulin resistance. This condition can increase the risk of developing Type 2 diabetes later in life. Obesity is another medical condition that can contribute to the development of diabetes. As mentioned earlier, excess body fat can cause the body to become insulin resistant, leading to high blood sugar levels. However, there is also evidence to suggest that obesity can cause the pancreas to produce less insulin, further exacerbating the issue. Obesity is a growing problem worldwide, and if left unchecked, it could lead to an increase in diabetes cases. Apart from the physical causes mentioned above, there are also psychological and emotional factors that can play a role in the development of diabetes mellitus. Chronic stress can cause an increase in the production of cortisol, a hormone that helps the body deal with stress. However, in excessive amounts, cortisol can interfere with the production and effectiveness of insulin, leading to a rise in blood sugar levels. Moreover, people who experience significant emotional distress or trauma may engage in unhealthy coping mechanisms, such as binge eating or substance abuse, which can also contribute to the development of diabetes.

chapter3

types diabetic mellitus

Type 1 diabetes, also known as insulin-dependent diabetes or juvenile diabetes, is an autoimmune disease where the immune system attacks and destroys the cells in the pancreas that produce insulin. Insulin is a hormone that helps regulate the levels of glucose in the blood. Without enough insulin, the body is unable to properly use glucose, leading to a buildup of sugar in the blood. This type of diabetes is usually diagnosed during childhood or adolescence, but it can occur at any age. The exact cause of Type 1 diabetes is still unknown, but it is believed to be a combination of genetic and environmental factors. People with a family history of Type 1 diabetes are at a higher risk of developing the disease. Certain viruses and infections have also been linked to the development of Type 1 diabetes. Symptoms of this type of diabetes may include increased thirst and urination, unexplained weight loss, extreme hunger, fatigue, and blurred vision. If left untreated, Type 1 diabetes can lead to serious health complications such as heart disease, nerve damage, kidney disease, and even vision loss. Type 1 diabetes is treated by replacing the missing insulin in the body through insulin injections or an insulin pump. Along with insulin therapy, individuals with Type 1 diabetes must also carefully monitor their blood sugar levels, follow a healthy diet plan, and engage in regular physical activity. It is important for people with Type 1 diabetes to maintain a consistent routine to keep their blood sugar levels under control. On the other hand, Type 2 diabetes, also known as non-insulin dependent diabetes, is the most common type of diabetes, accounting for about 90% of all cases. This type of diabetes occurs when the body becomes resistant to the effects of insulin, leading to high blood sugar levels. In the initial stages of Type 2 diabetes, the body may still produce enough insulin, but the cells in the body do not respond to it properly. Later on, the body may not produce enough insulin to meet the body's needs. The main risk factors for developing Type 2 diabetes include being overweight, having a sedentary lifestyle, and having a family history of the disease. Additionally, older age, race, ethnicity, and certain medical conditions such as polycystic ovary syndrome or prediabetes can increase the risk of developing Type 2 diabetes. Symptoms of this type of diabetes may be similar to those of Type 1, but they may develop gradually and go unnoticed for years. Some common symptoms include frequent urination, increased thirst, fatigue, blurred vision, and slow healing of wounds. Treatment for Type 2 diabetes usually involves lifestyle changes such as maintaining a healthy weight, following a balanced diet, and engaging in regular physical activity. In some cases, medication may also be prescribed to help manage blood sugar levels. Oral medications such as metformin, sulfonylureas, and thiazolidinediones can help increase insulin sensitivity or reduce glucose production in the liver. In more advanced cases, insulin therapy may be necessary to control blood sugar levels. Aside from these two main types of diabetes, there are also other less common types, including gestational diabetes, which occurs during pregnancy and can increase the risk of Type 2 diabetes later in life. Another type is maturity onset diabetes of the young (MODY), which is a rare genetic form of diabetes that affects people at a younger age and often runs in families. Managing diabetes requires constant monitoring of blood sugar levels, regular visits to healthcare professionals, and adherence to treatment plans. Blood sugar levels must be kept within a specific range to prevent both short-term and long-term complications.   Short-term complications of diabetes include hypoglycemia (low blood sugar) and hyperglycemia (high blood sugar), both of which can be dangerous if not treated promptly. In the long run, diabetes can lead to serious health complications such as heart disease, nerve damage, kidney disease, vision problems, and amputation. In addition to medical treatment, it is also important for individuals with diabetes to make necessary lifestyle changes to better manage the disease. This includes following a healthy diet that is low in sugar, salt, and saturated fats, quitting smoking, and maintaining a healthy weight. Regular physical activity is also essential in managing diabetes as it helps improve insulin sensitivity and cardiovascular health.

chapter4

diabetic mellitus ppt

Diabetes can be categorized into three main types: type 1 diabetes, type 2 diabetes, and gestational diabetes. Type 1 diabetes is an autoimmune disorder where the body's immune system attacks and destroys the cells in the pancreas that produce insulin. It is usually diagnosed in childhood or adolescence and requires lifelong insulin therapy. Type 2 diabetes, on the other hand, is the most common type and accounts for 90-95% of all diabetes cases. It is mainly caused by lifestyle factors such as obesity, physical inactivity, and unhealthy eating habits. In type 2 diabetes, the body becomes resistant to the effects of insulin, and the pancreas may also produce less insulin than needed. Gestational diabetes occurs during pregnancy when the mother's body is not able to produce enough insulin to meet the demands of pregnancy. It usually resolves after childbirth but increases the risk of developing type 2 diabetes later in life. The main symptoms of diabetes include frequent urination, increased thirst, extreme hunger, unexplained weight loss, fatigue, blurred vision, and slow healing of wounds. However, some people with type 2 diabetes may not experience any symptoms, and the disease is often diagnosed during routine medical check-ups. If left untreated, diabetes can lead to various serious complications, such as heart disease, stroke, kidney disease, nerve damage, and blindness. To diagnose diabetes, a doctor may recommend a series of tests, including blood sugar level tests, oral glucose tolerance test, glycated hemoglobin (A1C) test, and urine tests. These tests measure the levels of glucose in the blood and help determine the type of diabetes and the most suitable treatment plan. The primary treatment goal for diabetes is to control blood sugar levels and prevent or delay the onset of complications. Treatment options for diabetes vary depending on the type and severity of the disease but may include lifestyle changes, oral medications, and insulin therapy. Lifestyle changes, such as maintaining a healthy weight, exercising regularly, and following a healthy diet, are crucial in managing all types of diabetes. In some cases, oral medications, such as metformin, may be prescribed to help lower blood sugar levels. Insulin therapy is often necessary for people with type 1 diabetes and may be recommended for those with type 2 diabetes who are unable to control their blood sugar levels with oral medications. One of the key components of managing diabetes is self-care. People with diabetes need to regularly monitor their blood sugar levels, take medications as prescribed, follow a healthy meal plan, and keep track of their physical activity. They also need to be aware of the signs and symptoms of high or low blood sugar levels, as well as the proper steps to take to bring their levels back to a normal range. Self-care also involves regularly visiting a healthcare professional for check-ups, screenings, and adjustments to the treatment plan as needed. It is essential to understand that managing diabetes is not just about controlling blood sugar levels. People with diabetes also need to manage other risk factors for complications, such as high blood pressure and high cholesterol levels. This may involve taking medication to control blood pressure and cholesterol levels and making necessary lifestyle changes. The importance of education and awareness in managing diabetes cannot be overstated. To effectively manage their disease, individuals with diabetes must have a good understanding of the disease and its management. Diabetes education programs, either individually or in a group setting, provide people with the knowledge and skills necessary to manage their condition and prevent complications. These programs cover topics such as monitoring blood sugar levels, healthy eating, physical activity, and medication management. In recent years, technology has played an essential role in diabetes management. Continuous glucose monitoring (CGM) devices, insulin pumps, and smartphone applications are among the many technological advancements that have significantly improved the lives of people with diabetes. CGM devices continuously measure glucose levels and provide real-time readings, helping individuals make informed decisions about their diet, exercise, and insulin dosing. Insulin pumps deliver insulin continuously, mimicking the functions of a healthy pancreas, while smartphone applications help track blood sugar levels, food intake, and physical activity. An important aspect of diabetes management is maintaining a healthy diet. People with diabetes should aim to follow a balanced diet that includes a variety of fruits, vegetables, whole grains, lean proteins, and healthy fats while limiting saturated and trans fats, added sugars, and sodium. Portion control is also crucial, as excess weight and obesity are significant risk factors for type 2 diabetes. Registered dietitians can help individuals with diabetes plan and manage their meals to achieve the right balance of nutrients and calories. Exercise is another crucial component of diabetes management. Physical activity helps lower blood sugar levels, reduce the risk of heart disease, and improve overall health. Regular exercise also helps with weight management, which is essential for people with diabetes. Individuals with diabetes should aim for at least 150 minutes of moderate-intensity aerobic exercise, such as brisk walking, per week. They should also incorporate strength training activities at least twice a week to build muscle mass and improve insulin sensitivity.

The end